Alkaline Diet

The Ultimate Beginner's Alkaline Diet Food Guide to Naturally Reclaim & Balance Your Health, Achieve Rapid Weight Loss, Understand pH and Transform Your Body + Fresh, Fast & Delicious Recipes Included!

By *Simone Jacobs*

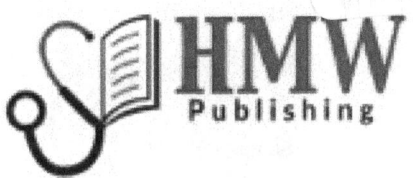

For more great books visit:

HMWPublishing.com

Get another book for Free

I want to thank you for purchasing this book and offer you another book (just as long and valuable as this book), "Health & Fitness Mistakes You Don't Know You're Making", completely free.

Visit the link below to signup and receive it:

www.hmwpublishing.com/gift

In this book, I will break down the most common health & fitness mistakes, you are probably committing right now, and I will reveal how you can easily get in the best shape of your life!

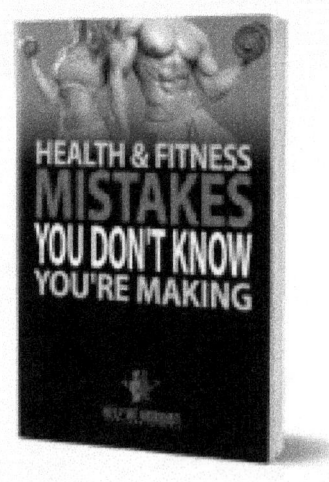

In addition to this valuable gift, you will also have an opportunity to get our new books for free, enter giveaways, and receive other valuable emails from me. Again, visit the link to sign up:

www.hmwpublishing.com/gift

Table of Contents

Introduction 1

    Dash Notes To The Ash Diet – What Is It Exactly? 3

Chapter 1: Acid-Alkaline Balance 101 - All The Gist You Need To Know About pH and What It Has To Do With Your Health? 5

    Health and pH 6

    Determining What Affects Your pH 8

        Stimulants 9

        Exercise 10

        Stress 11

        Water 12

    Personalizing Your Plan 13

        Assess Your pH Tendencies (Some People Are Naturally Acidic) 13

Chapter 2: Acidic Wastes and How High Acid Levels Cause Diseases and Overweight 18

    Claim to Bone Loss Due to High Acid Diets 19

    Claim to Kidney Stones Due to High Acid Diet ... 19

    Claim to Cancer Due to High Acid Diets 20

    When They Say High Acid = High Weight Gain .. 22

Chapter 3: Symptoms of Having a Low Alkaline Level 24

    Heartburn and GERD 24

    Tooth Decay 27

Blood Sugar Imbalance 28

Chapter 4: Treatment of Acidosis 30

Chapter 5: Benefits of the Alkaline Diet 32

Preserves Bone Density and Promotes Muscle Mass 34

Lowers Risk of Hypertension and Stroke 35

Helps Enhance Immune Function 36

Aids in Lowering Cancer Risk 36

Lowers Chronic Pain and Inflammation 37

Improves Vitamin and Mineral Absorption 39

Maintains Optimal Weight 40

Chapter 6: Good Alkaline Food and Bad Alkaline Food 41

Food to avoid 41

Food to eat to increase alkalinity 43

Bonus Chapter: Delicious Alkalinizing Recipes 46

1. Tomatoes with Quinoa Filling 46
2. High Protein Blueberry Spinach Smoothie 49
3. Minty Banana Coconut Shake 51
4. Lettuce Cups filled with Adzuki Beans and Avocado 53
5. Lentil and Thyme Soup 55
6. Cucumber Lavender Water 57
7. Watermelon Mint Water 58
8. Chilled Watercress With Avocado and Cucumber Soup 59

9. Green Curry 61
10. Chocolate Mousse with Avocado 63
11. Veggie Sticks with Guacamole Dip 64
12. Naked Chilli 66
13. Kale with Quinoa Salad Served with Lemon Vinaigrette Dressing 69
14. Berry Almond Smoothie 71
15. Banana Almond Berry Smoothie 73
16. Veggie Carrot and Leeks Soup 74
17. Veggie Delight Pasta 76
18. Brussels Sprouts Salad with Pistachios and Lemon 79
19. Pasta Zucchini with Spinach Lemon Pesto 81
20. Sweet Potato Soup With a Hint of Curry .. 83
21. Alkaline Power Up Treats 85
22. Choco Mint Smoothie 87
23. Detoxifying Ginger Lemon Turmeric Tea . 89

Conclusion 91

Final Words 93

About the Co-Author 94

INTRODUCTION

Recently, massive attention is directed towards Alkaline Diet, as well as a surprising increase in the number of people getting to the bottom of what it is and what makes it so accessible. Most importantly, how efficient it can be to heal your body. In fact, the increased popularity of Alkaline Diet is so impressive that it has resulted in a lot of literature. A quick Google search of "Alkaline Diet" would return 3.18 million results on the topic in a split second. That being said, which writing should you focus your attention? Which ones are worth your time? And which ones would give you the unbiased information you need (without all the hullabaloos and hard to understand science jargons)?

Well, you have made the right decision in picking up this book *"Alkaline Diet: The Ultimate Beginner's Alkaline Diet Food Guide to Naturally Reclaim & Balance Your Health, Achieve Rapid Weight Loss, Understand pH and Transform Your Body + 50 Delicious Recipes."*

This book will walk you through all the essential facts you need to know about the Alkaline Diet. All the necessary things without the hard to comprehend nonsense. Just pure, practical information along with straightforward to follow suggestions on getting into the diet as well as quick fix recipes to get you started with your best foot forward. You will get to learn the importance of a well maintained alkaline digestive system and better appreciate a lifestyle of eating healthily without having to sacrifice a lot. Not only will this book provide you will all the helpful tips to get you started, but will also give you advice as to how to keep maintaining the alkaline diet to ensure your success. The bonus fifty simple recipes will help get you started right away. You don't get a better deal than that!

Also, before you get started, I recommend you **joining our email newsletter** to receive updates on any upcoming new book releases or promotions. You can sign-up for free, and as a bonus, you will receive a free gift. Our "*Health & Fitness Mistakes You Don't Know You're Making*" book! This book has been written to demystify, expose the top do's and don'ts and to finally equip you with the information you need to get in the best shape of your life. Due to the overwhelming amount of mis-information and lies told by magazines and self-proclaimed "gurus", it's becoming harder and harder to get reliable information to get in shape. As opposed to having to go through dozens of biased, unreliable and untrustworthy sources to get your health & fitness information. Everything you need to help you has been broken down in this book for you to easily follow and to immediately get results to achieve your desired fitness goals in the shortest amount of time.

Once again, to join our free email newsletter and to receive a free copy of this valuable book, please visit the link and signup now: www.hmwpublishing.com/gift

Dash Notes To The Ash Diet – What Is It Exactly?

To put it simply, the Alkaline Diet or the Ash Diet is a form of diet where you consume food that will encourage the formation of alkaline rich products in the body. This diet allows for the slight increase in pH within the system to support and promote a healthier system within the body. As it has been shown that your internal pH is affected by the mineral composition of the food you consume, the rationale of Alkaline Diet is to promote the ingestion of food that will help balance the pH levels of the fluids in our body. Since abnormal pH levels in the body have been linked to disease and illnesses, the idea is by following an alkaline diet we balance our pH and prevent chronic diseases from occurring.

Chapter 1: Acid-Alkaline Balance 101 - All The Gist You Need To Know About pH and What It Has To Do With Your Health?

To better understand how the Alkaline Diet works, it is essential that we first dig into the science that backs it up. I know I have said previously that this book will shy away from all the science gibberish, but I assure you this couldn't be any more simple than your typical high school class. We first need to know how pH balance works. The pH scale which is a numerical measure of a solution's acidity or basicity runs from 1 to 14. Seven would be considered the neutral ground and anything below the seven value is deemed to be acidic while anything above it is alkaline or basic. The human body is highly dependent upon an optimal pH where specific regions or systems has strictly controlled mechanisms to maintain this optimal pH. In fact, much of our bodily functions are so heavily dependent on pH that a slight deviation in the optimal pH range could result in catastrophic results, and in some instances even possibly death. And we're not talking about 2 or 5 point change here, it could be as little a deviation as 0.2-0.5 from the optimal range, and that could mean a life or death situation.

When It comes to human digestion, it is the kidneys that would be in charge of maintaining the pH of the blood very close to a value of 7.4 by either secreting or absorbing specific compounds to regulate the pH. This is the main reason that the system does not support bug down if we suddenly ingested a highly acidic diet, the kidney serves to provide the pH buffering mechanism. However, research has been consistent in showing that a chronic diet of highly acidic food could take its toll in the human body and eventually, over time, this may lead to some health consequences.

Health and pH

What exactly happens to the human body when the pH is not ideal? First of all, if the pH of the body tends to vary a lot, essential proteins in the body which we call enzymes are affected gravely. Enzymes in the body are responsible for making indispensable reactions to take place, and they can only function in the optimal pH. Whenever they are exposed to either a pH so much higher or so much lower than their optimal pH, the enzymes tend to change its structure and cease to function. This can be disastrous to the body because then we will be inhibiting a lot of required biological functions.

Another importance of a balanced internal pH is protection against microbial pathogens, the bacterial, fungal and viral microorganisms we call germs and continuously invade our bodies. These living organisms to thrive under their optimal pH. Our bodies have been designed to function well under a specific pH, anything below or above that will allow these invasive microorganisms to flourish in our body.

And one other important feature about optimal pH is the condition of the immune system. The immune system consists of an army of white blood cells and other cells designed to engulf and rid our bodies of any threat. These immune system cells are highly dependent on the body's alkalinity or acidity that anything beyond the optimal pH will compromise our immune system and hinder it from performing functionally.

To be able to maintain the slightly central state, the body needs to be in constant work at releasing or absorbing compounds. Most of the reactions naturally occurring within the human body lead to the formation of acidic compounds and the body needs to adjust to that immediately. This condition is further perturbed if we burden our bodies with acid-producing foods in our diet time and time again.

Determining What Affects Your pH

pH is not only determined by the diet that you chose to maintain or even the type of food that you ingest. This condition, like most everything when it comes to a human being's wellness, is also heavily dependent on the holistic lifestyle of the person. Just like everything that is related to health (or more broadly to life), moderation is key. Balance in everything is the solution to keeping a fit physical, emotional and mental physique. Too much of something is just as bad as having too little of one thing. Furthermore, the proper pH would be variable for particular regions throughout your body. A phenomenon that is highly reasonable, given that not all organs would function in much the same way and each intricate process in the human body is involving a lot of sophisticated methods – for this book, we would focus on how pH in our digestive system would affect your wellness. The following factors are some of the most common that would change your digestive system's pH considerably.

Stimulants

The stomach and gastrointestinal tract is a complex system, and to function well in digesting our food intake into smaller molecules that would be more meaningful for nutrient uptake of the body; it needs to be in the proper pH range. Several factors stimulate the secretion of acid in the gastrointestinal tract, and most of these are dependent on things we ingest in our body.

When it comes to acid secretion, high-protein food is more effective stimulants in the body compared to food that is mostly made up of starchy products, carbohydrates or lipids. This means that ingesting high protein nuts, beans, eggs, and meat would better spike up the gastrointestinal tract's acidity than reaching for food that is mostly bread, sugar or fatty food.

Exercise

Exercise has been shown to positively improve the efficacy of digestion and eventually lead to a healthy weight. Different types of training could lead to mixed results and negative impacts on the digestive system. For instance, cardio exercises such as running on a treadmill or riding a bike can help reduce or avoid heartburn occurrences. It has been shown that low impact exercises that promote proper breathing and heart rate can encourage a more healthy bowel movement.

On the other hand, extreme exercises that usually involve high impact and repetitive movements such as heavy bench presses or hanging leg raises or barbell squats could bring more harm than help by causing digestive disorders. Thus it is vital that exercise should also be taken in moderation.

Stress

There is an intricate relationship between the digestive system and the nervous system where the nervous system could have an elaborate control over the functions of the digestive system, and mostly involving the secretion of hydrochloric acid in the stomach. This is the reason why your stomach would be triggered to secrete acid in preparation for a meal as soon as you see, imagine or smell food. This kind of stimulation is not dependent on the food but is mostly dependent on the nervous system's perception. In this same way, stress, where high levels of stress hormones are released in the body, could also profoundly affect the acidity of the stomach and eventually every part of the digestive system. Stress can cause the shut down of the digestive system because the central nervous system shuts down as well. This decreases secretion in the digestive system and eventually the inflammation of the gastrointestinal system, making the body all the more susceptible to infection.

To aid in digestion, we must always keep our stress levels in check and under control. Relaxation therapies are available for dealing with stress issues, and quite possibly the best means to deal with stress is to limit altogether or avoid the cause of stress.

Water

The common conception is that water would dilute digestive juices. This is a reasonable notion, given that water is the universal solvent. Water aids in the proper digestion of food, but by itself, it cannot prompt absorption. However, the intake of ionized or alkalinized water is a different aspect. It has been said that ionized water has had established effects that promote proper digestion but only not within 20 minutes of a meal, this includes before and after ingestion. This is because it has been shown that the high levels of ions in the alkaline water could interfere with the acidity of the digestive system and this, in turn, would cause problems with food digestion.

On the one hand, drinking alkaline water before or after the 20-minute time frame is thought to be good practice for a more healthy digestive tract.

Personalizing Your Plan

With all the advantages of keeping a healthy pH, it is highly necessary that we know how to keep up with our acidity or alkalinity. The trick is knowing that not everybody type is the same so each of our bodies would react to a particular trigger differently. In the following section, we will be learning about how easy it is to measure our body's pH and then we will learn some practical tips about how to assess our pH tendencies.

Assess Your pH Tendencies (Some People Are Naturally Acidic)

It is highly essential that we test our body's pH because it will not only give us a sense of where our body is in the pH zone. It will also get a clue whether it is gearing towards metabolic acidity, or balance, or is more alkaline than what is to be expected as optimal for our body type.

The best, and possibly most straightforward and most

practical, a method for determining your body's pH is to test for your body's excreted fluids like saliva or urine. All you need to have to decide this is a way to measure it. Now, there is the more sophisticated way of measuring pH where you use laboratory grade equipment called a pH meter that would have this probe that you need to dip into your solution of interest for you to be able to quantify the pH as accurately as possible. Fortunately for us, we don't have to go through all the complexity and suddenly feel like we're going into our high school science lab again. Luckily, we can use a tool as simple as paper.

pH papers are available pieces of documents that have been designed specifically for the detection of pH. It would have all these indicators that would change a different color depending on the acidity or basicity of your liquid. All you have to do is wet this pH paper with your solution, wait a couple of seconds and compare the color change in the strip of pH paper with the indicated pH value.

In testing our body's present pH state, it is best that you perform this test in the morning before you have taken your breakfast to record your body's steady state pH without the influence of food yet. So, do this test the first thing in your morning routine after you wake up – and as much as possible, when you have had a good restful sleep of at least 6 hours, this is to make sure that stress is not affecting your pH readings.

To do this test using urine samples, you could collect your morning's first urine in a cup and dip the strip of pH paper to determine your body's pH. Another option is to do the test using your saliva. Among the two samples, research has shown that the former is better, especially if the urine sample is the first one released after at least six hours of sleep. Saliva is less adequate just because there are a lot more enzymes in the saliva sample and also because urine samples would be coming directly from inside of the body.

To test your pH using saliva samples – again, note that this is best done using samples taken first thing in the morning – take a mouthful of water and gargle and rinse your mouth with it. Spit out the wash and then collect some of your salivae using a spoon. Dip the pH paper strip into the sample of saliva and wait for the color to change and stabilize. It is essential that you do not brush your teeth, eat or drink anything yet before you perform the test, remember we are trying to establish your body's present pH.

Do these simple tests to monitor your body's pH. Although you do not need to measure your pH daily, it would be nice to incorporate this simple morning routine into one of your weekends. Do this test once or twice a week and keep a record of your pH changes. It is especially important if you have the goal in mind to control your body's pH – which I assume would be your case since you are now holding this book in your hand.

Also, an important note is that while others, more often than the other, may start out with an acidic pH with values lower than 6.5, this is entirely normal. Especially given the kind of diet an average American would have nowadays. All you have to do is increase your pH by increasing your intake of fruits and vegetables, nuts, root crops, spices and seeds and all in the effort of improving your alkalinity. Lucky for you, this book will help you achieve that with a lot of practical tips and easy to make recipes.

On the other hand, if your pH is above the 7.5 mark, suggesting highly alkaline steady-state pH then this could be due to high levels of nitrogen in your urine or saliva sample. This is observed when there is more than the usual catabolism or the natural breakdown of specific body tissues. The benefit of having to measure your body's pH routinely is for you to at least keep track of your body's changes. If your readings have been consistently close to the 8.0 pH mark, then you should contact your health professional and seek advice as to how to manage tissue repair and avoid the too much catabolic state in your body.

Chapter 2: Acidic Wastes and How High Acid Levels Cause Diseases and Overweight

Nutrition plays a lead role in the overall wealth of a person, and taking in the wrong kinds of food could lead to deterioration of the human body. We need to be very careful with how we take care of our bodies because despite it's millions of years of evolutionary advantage and learning to cope with any attack there is, our bodies are still very much susceptible to harm. And the most efficient and most silent attacker to our health is the food we intake. We might not be aware, but the little by little amounts of greasy fries, or slimy burger patties or burning alcohol may be enough to accumulate and eat up through our systems.

When it comes to highly acidic diets and its link to some diseases, here are just a few of the most significant impacts acidic diets do to our bodies:

Claim to Bone Loss Due to High Acid Diets

When you have too much acid within your system, you tend to develop chronic acidosis, and this disease has been linked in many studies to bone diseases due to decrease in bone density. Too much of the acid, highly abundant in proton molecules in the body, in the blood, would mean that your body would tend to compensate for this pH drop by attempting to increase it. And the way the body responds to it is by releasing calcium ions from the bones into the blood. Calcium ions are rare alkaline minerals. Having chronic acidosis, however, would tend to deplete the bones from the much-needed calcium they need to establish bone density and this, in turn, results in bone loss and diseases.

Claim to Kidney Stones Due to High Acid Diet

It has been shown that people who are suffering from a chronic kidney disease could have a higher risk of their disease progressing into and eventually developing into kidney failure when they routinely have highly acidic diets. High acid diets are rich in meats and have been linked to this progression to kidney failures. In fact, chronic kidney disease patients have three times higher risk of developing kidney failure as compared to their high alkaline consuming counterparts. People should pay more attention to this tendency, especially if they are already at a risk of kidney diseases.

Claim to Cancer Due to High Acid Diets

There have been a sufficient amount of data out there that would provide the link between pH and cancer. In papers published, they would present researchers that support how cancer would thrive in an acidic environment. This is as a result of cancer cells releasing too much lactic acid, in contrast, it is in the acidic environment that cancer cells would start to have a more significant chance of reproducing. Studies say that as the body begins to accumulate acid-forming substances, the body starts to release materials that would try to circumvent the drop in pH. Over time these elements become toxic to the cell as oxygen levels drop, and the hereditary DNA and respiratory enzymes start getting affected. The natural tendency of the battery is to enter into the physical cell death or apoptosis since the cells are no longer beneficial to the body, they are more of a liability than an asset. However, some cells survive, and instead of entering into normal cell suicide would become abnormal cells having the ability to withstand high levels of acid substances in its environment. The abnormal cells become what we know as malignant cells that are no longer responding to the nervous system, nor to the body's control of gene expression of its DNA. So instead, these cancerous cells start reproducing and making more and more copies of itself, growing indefinitely and without and control until it has become cancer. That silent killer that is devastating millions of the world's population now.

When They Say High Acid = High Weight Gain

There is an intricate relationship between the body's fat and the body's acidity. Although this fact seems to escape a lot of people, putting all the blame into the well marked "culprit" fat, it may be, so that body acidity has much to do with a person's body weight, or maybe even be the mastermind culprit after all. So how do we make sense of this? Wait a minute, isn't obesity measured by the excess amount of fat you have after all? So it is right to blame it all on the fat!

Well, not entirely true. The thing is when your body is experiencing too much acidity; it starts to produce all these toxins that are profoundly harmful to the body. As we've seen above it can lead to bone loss diseases, kidney failures or cancer. It has even been linked to premature aging, diabetes and a lot of other problems. In response to this possible threat, the body tries to protect itself by creating fat cells that would serve as storage vessels for these toxins, absorbing the excess acidic substances and preventing it from further causing harm to the body. It follows that the more acidic materials the body produces, the more fat cells will be needed to store these toxins.

So, in a nutshell, the best way to look at this is if you do not have a lot of junk that you have to store then there would not have to be a lot of these large compartments. To begin with, If you did not have a lot of the harmful acidic substances that act as toxins, then your body would not need to produce more fats. So maybe the next time you start pinpointing at your fats for giving you a horrible time trying to fit into your jeans from last year, maybe start looking at the real cause of the problem and kickstart at rethinking your diet.

Chapter 3: Symptoms of Having a Low Alkaline Level

Heartburn and GERD

Heartburn is one of the most common medical problems that Americans are experiencing on a monthly basis, up to 40% of Americans report to suffer from this condition regularly. It has become part of an average American's lifestyle that one would easily shrug off the problem as soon as it persists thinking that it is merely one of those days where you had something "bad" to eat. As soon as that burning and scorching acidic sensation broils inside your chest, the first go-to treatment of any ordinary American would be a quick discomfort relief – the most popular being the handy Pepto-Bismol. But heartburns should not be shrugged off quickly, the underlying reason for having these heartburns may be more severe than you think and more so if the problem persists more frequently than usual.

The burning sensation one feels as a result of heartburn is

caused by the reflux of acid-laden contents in the stomach as a consequence of having a faulty esophageal valve that keeps contents of the stomach from coming back up. Heartburn is the primary and noticeable side effect of low alkaline diet, and this can lead to a number other more life-threatening problems to a person.

The more severe form of heartburn is called Gastroesophageal Reflux Disease or GERD; this occurs when an individual is experiencing chronic heartburns, and uncontrolled persistence of this disease can lead to significant health issues that could damage your teeth and esophagus.

The esophagus links your mouth to your stomach, and when acid from the stomach flows back up, this sets the stage for swelling and irritation of the esophageal lining. The inflammation can make it very hard for a person to swallow and is a health condition called esophagitis.

On the one hand, when GERD continues to persist it will eventually cause sores in the epidermal walls of the esophagus, this makes GERD the leading cause of ulcers.

Associated symptoms of esophageal ulcers could include chest pain, nausea along with the pain accompanied by swallowing.

When inflammation obstinately continues, over time the swelling can lead to permanent damage and eventual scarring of the esophageal lining. Building up of this scar tissue in the esophagus would narrow the esophageal tube and create constricted regions called the esophageal strictures. These make it even harder to swallow food and liquids which eventually leads to weight loss and dehydration. This is a severe problem and should not be taken lightly. Treatments include a procedure that helps loosen the strictures by gently stretching the esophagus.

One other serious problem associated with acid reflux is called Barrett's esophagus, and about 1 out of 10 people with GERD develop this condition. This issue is caused by stomach acid making precancerous changes in the epidermal (outer or surface lining) cells of the esophagus. This increases the risk for esophageal cancer, luckily only 1 out of a hundred people with Barrett's esophagus was found to have esophageal cancer. Still, this should not be taken for granted since the condition does not lead to any apparent symptoms and chest pains which are usually associated with esophageal cancer typically appear only in later stages of the disease when it has progressed. It is nevertheless best to seek professional advice if you have had more than the usual bouts of acid refluxes and heartburns recently. To be able to rule out cancer for certain, endoscopy may be needed wherein a thin, flexible tube with a camera at the tip and linked to the computer enables a health professional to view the insides of your esophagus.

Tooth Decay

This symptom is mostly related to the above condition of having acid flow back into your mouth from the stomach. Heartburns as a result of low alkaline diet can also take a levy on your dashing smile. Stomach acid, like most acid, is highly corrosive and can wear down the teeth's hard outer covering that serves as a protective layer called enamel. The enamel gives us our pearly white smiles and helps us prevent plaque buildup and cavities, without it the teeth weakens and turns yellow.

Blood Sugar Imbalance

Some symptoms associated with sugar imbalance as a result of low pH levels include stubborn headaches that would only go away after eating. Also, there are bouts of energy swings during the day where you may start out with such a high energy and switch to being too tired and over fatigued in a matter of hours without even exerting too much effort. Low pH levels could also increase cravings for simple sugars, carbohydrates and loads of sweets as this provides immediate relief to sugar discomfort. There are also those episodes of blocking out or zoning out after a meal or what millennials like to call "food coma." Coffee addicts may have to beware of their dependence on coffee may also be due to low alkalinity. And lightheadedness could also result in an effect of missing meals.

The imbalance of sugar in the body is a result of your body

not being able to handle its fuel source – glucose – efficiently. For proper function, the body needs to metabolize, digest and break down glucose and maintain blood glucose levels at an optimal range. Anything below this may cause lightheadedness as this provides less glucose to the brain especially. On the one hand, having too much glucose would lead to what we call "sugar rush" where a person experiences episodes of high energy vents. The fluctuation is getting too high energy swings during or after a meal to very low energy swings when you skip a meal, and your body runs out of its food reserve.

CHAPTER 4: TREATMENT OF ACIDOSIS

To accurately correct the real cause of the problem, the doctor needs to be able to determine the patient's condition and only then can he or she be able to provide with the right kind of treatment for acidosis. There are however some temporary immediate relief treatments that can be used for any types of acidosis regardless of what causes it. One of the most popular treatment is the oral ingestion of sodium bicarbonate (baking soda or generically known pharmaceutically as an antacid). This will help increase the blood pH temporarily and is a preferred go to drug as it can be purchased over the counter and can be taken in orally or some forms can be done via an intravenous (IV) drip.

Acidosis that are affecting the respiratory tract can be treated by targeting the airways and provide relief to the lungs. Drugs designed to dilate the airways can be prescribed, or devices that enable a patient that has obstructed breathing or weakened respiratory muscles to breathe better can also be given to a patient. Devices such as these are called CPAP (Continuous Positive Airway Pressure) devices.

Acidosis that have been associated with kidney failure could also be treated explicitly with sodium citrate to help ease problems with kidney stones. Improper blood sugar balance that results from pH imbalance could be treated with IV fluids and insulin to maintain pH levels to the optimum; this is especially necessary for patients already suffering from diabetes mellitus or ketoacidosis.

Chapter 5: Benefits of the Alkaline Diet

Many types of research would continue to support the many benefits of taking in alkaline inducing diets. In fact, research has shown that from our early ancestors, a lot has considerably changed with our diet coming from a hunter-gathering system to our present condition where the majority of our food intake now would consist of fast food choices and high sodium and high-fat content. Average food intake from hundreds of years past used to be high in potassium, magnesium, and chloride. Until the uprising of the agricultural revolution where humans need not move around to hunt for their food anymore, and instead, they have learned to grow and care for their food. And then followed by the mass industrialization where food businesses would start to improve and people would rely on other businesses to serve their food instead. This shift up to today has increased the sodium intake of people.

Typically it would be the task of our kidneys to help maintain this electrolyte imbalance or shift − electrolytes such as the magnesium, calcium, potassium, and sodium. When the body is dealing with high acidity, the body will use these electrolytes to fight against bitterness.

Whereas potassium used to outnumber sodium in an average human's diet, this has now dramatically shifter to almost threefold. Increasing in sodium would mean that we have less of the required electrolytes, antioxidants, essential vitamins and fiber to ward off or level out the acidity. To top it all off, the typical diet of the western world is concentrated with refined fats, sodium, simple sugars and chloride.

All of these changes have inevitably led to an increase in metabolic acidosis, a condition where the pH levels of the human body are no longer optimal. Many are now suffering from a deficient nutrient intake, with micronutrient deficiencies for potassium and magnesium.

Metabolic acidosis increases the aging process and would eventually lead to gradual loss of organ functions and degeneration of bone mass and many tissues.

On the one hand, there is still hope because the effects of highly acidic substances in the body could be very simply reversed by changing our diets and rethinking about how we treat food consumption.

If the risks of having highly acidic internal body system will not persuade you enough to enter into an alkaline diet, then this following list of the benefits of alkaline diets would hopefully, finally, do the trick.

Preserves Bone Density and Promotes Muscle Mass

The development and maintenance of bone structure are highly dependent on the intake of minerals. A myriad of researchers has linked the consumption of more alkalizing vegetables and fruits to a better response of the body in protecting against decreased bone strength and muscle wasting as the body continues to age. This wasting of the body's muscle and bones is a condition called sarcopenia.

An alkaline diet helps to balance the ratios of minerals necessary and crucial for bone building and lean muscle mass maintenance. These minerals include not only the well-known calcium but magnesium and phosphate as well.

Alkaline diet not only helps in mineral balance, but it also helps improve the production of growth hormones and vitamin D absorption. These biomolecules are essential players that help protect bone loss and also contribute heavily to lessening many other chronic diseases.

Lowers Risk of Hypertension and Stroke

One of the well-known effects of engaging in an alkaline diet is the response to anti-aging, and the diet does this by decreasing inflammation in the body, consequently increasing the production of growth hormones. Increase in growth hormone and reduction in inflammation has been shown to improve cardiovascular health by preventing a lot of the commonly reported problems such as hypertension caused by high blood pressure, high cholesterol content, stroke, kidney stones and even memory loss.

Helps Enhance Immune Function

The body's first defense to get rid of harmful elements in the body is to properly dispose of them as wastes, expel them out of the body or convert them into less toxic substances. However, when the body, particularly the cells, lack enough of the crucial minerals that would help them perform this function, the entire body would suffer. The absorption of vitamins is hugely compromised by the loss of essential minerals. As a result, toxins and pathogens (germs such as bacteria, virus or fungi) start to accumulate in the body and as a result systematically weaken the immune system.

Aids in Lowering Cancer Risk

A lot of peer-reviewed research publications have shown that cancerous cell death, or the condition we technically call apoptosis, was more likely to occur in a body that is high in alkalinity. This proves that this links cancer prevention to a high alkaline diet. Indeed, the process of preventing cancer development is now believed to be connected with a shift in pH towards a more alkaline end due to an alteration in the electric charges and the release of basic components of proteins. Not only is an alkaline diet beneficial for people who have not yet developed cancer by lowering their risk for it. An alkaline diet has also been shown to provide people being treated for cancer or recovering from its treatments, with a better chance of ridding themselves of it. An alkaline diet has been shown to be more beneficial for a lot of chemotherapeutic chemicals and drugs that usually need a higher pH for it to work more efficiently.

Lowers Chronic Pain and Inflammation

Still much more other studies have revealed the link between a high pH diet with that of reduced levels of chronic pain. On the one hand, constant acidosis has been found to contribute to a lot of chronic pain disorders such as muscle spasms, chronic back pain, menstrual cramps, headaches, joint pains, and inflammation.

One significant study that has been performed by experts in Germany has shown that supplementing alkalinity to some patients suffering from chronic back pain in four weeks have shown a substantial decrease in pain for seventy-six out of eighty-two patients involved in the study. Although the mechanism for this preventive action has not yet been fully elucidated, apparently the link is there for a better lifestyle with the alkaline diet.

Improves Vitamin and Mineral Absorption

Magnesium is an essential systematic cofactor for thousands of enzymes required to perform some metabolic processes. The increase in magnesium content is therefore beneficial for a lot of bodily processes. Many people are, unfortunately, suffering from magnesium deficiency and mostly due to the choice in diet. The consequences of this lack are heart complications, headaches, muscle pains, anxiety and sleep disorders. Magnesium is one of the crucial elements required for vitamin D activation, necessary for the overall immune and endocrine function of the body.

Magnesium is present in a bulk of highly alkalinizing food, and thus just by increasing this food intake, you are already doing your body a tremendous amount of favor.

Maintains Optimal Weight

Limiting the intake of highly acid forming foods and instead shifting to higher consumption of more alkaline forming food can protect you from developing obesity. This is by decreasing the number of leptin levels in the body as well as inflammation. Leptin affects a person's cravings and is usually the culprit being blamed for why we reach for a second serving almost instantly after a meal. Inflammation and leptin levels also affect the body's fat burning abilities. Daily intake of the anti-inflammatory alkaline inducing foods would allow your body to reach normal leptin levels and help you fell satisfied and full easily and longer. Preventing you from overeating and only reaching for the right amount of calories you really need.

Chapter 6: Good Alkaline Food and Bad Alkaline Food

Food to avoid

Here are some of the food you need to eat less of if you find out that your pH is lower than the normal range. These food increase acidity and should be taken sparingly.

- Carbonated or soft drinks (soda)
- Dairy products such as cheese (especially parmesan and sharper cheese), milk and yogurt
- Simple Sugars
- Simple carbohydrates such as white bread, rice, and pasta
- Meat (Pork, chicken, beef, lamb) and fish – these should be taken in moderation

- Grains such as oats, cornmeal, wheat, rye, bran and spelt

- Grain products such as cereals, pastries, crackers

- Unsprouted beans (sprouted beans are alkaline forming foods): mung, navy, lentils, garbanzo, white, red, adzuki, broad

- Sunflower and pumpkin seeds

- Nuts such as pecans, walnuts, cashews, macadamias, pistachios, peanuts and brazil nuts

- Alcoholic beverages

- Caffeinated drinks

- Sweeteners (artificial or natural like barley syrup, honey, maple syrup, molasses, fructose)

- Soy sauce and table salt

- Mustard, ketchup, and mayonnaise

- White vinegar

Food to eat to increase alkalinity

These alkalinizing food list will help you neutralize the effects of eating foods that lower pH.

Here are some of the most common ones:

- Vegetables (practically all of this product are alkalinizing)

- Fruits (interestingly citrus fruits (rich in ascorbic acid or vitamin C and citric acid) are alkalinizing, only avoid cranberries, blueberries, prunes, and plums)

- Beans (especially sprouted ones) such as soy, green, lima, string and snap

- Peas

- Potatoes

- Exotic grains such as quinoa, millet, flax, and amaranth

- Nuts such as almonds and chestnuts

- Sprouted seeds of radish, chia, and alfalfa

- Unsalted butter
- Eggs
- Whey
- Herbal teas
- Garlic
- Cayenne pepper
- Gelatin
- Miso
- Vanilla spices
- Brewer's yeast
- Cold-processed and unprocessed oils

It is important to note that just because they are acid-forming, they should not be avoided altogether, in fact, many of these acid-forming food are necessary for healthy metabolism and proper body function. The key to utilizing this list of different pH regulating food is to know when to eat one kind sparingly and know when to eat more of the other. Again the most important thing when it comes to diet and health is the balance. The following chapter will help you appreciate the alkaline diet better with some fun and simple recipes that help give you the best out of your food selections.

BONUS CHAPTER: DELICIOUS ALKALINIZING RECIPES

1. Tomatoes with Quinoa Filling

SERVINGS: 4

INGREDIENTS

4 large tomatoes

2 cups quinoa seeds

6 cups baby spinach

4 cloves of garlic, minced

1 can kidney beans (rinse and drain)

¼ cup basil, (cut into thin strips)

2 tbsp. coconut oil

4 cups water

sea salt

black pepper to taste

PREPARATION

Turn on oven and set to 375 degrees, allow to reach temperature. Empty the insides of the tomatoes by making about a quarter inch slice on the top of the tomato and scooping out the inside contents with a spoon. Make a small cut off the bottom of the tomato to allow it to sit flat on a baking pan (Make sure not to cut too thick and ruin you're hollowed out tomatoes). Drizzle a little salt into the insides of the tomatoes.

Combine 4 cups of water with the quinoa seeds and cook the quinoa in a pot set on top of the stove on high heat. Allow the water to come to a boil and turn the heat down to the minimum setting and cover the pot. Keep cooking the quinoa seeds for an additional 30-45 minutes.

In another pan set on top of the medium heat, drizzle the coconut oil and fry garlic until it is lightly browned. Pour in the kidney beans into the pan and using a spatula, slightly crush them on the pan. Allow the beans to cook for about 1 -2 minutes. Pour in the baby spinach and as soon as they cook and wilt, add the basil. Season with salt and pepper.

In a large bowl, pour in your spinach mixture and cooked quinoa seeds. Carefully stuff your spinach-quinoa filling into your hollowed-out tomatoes. Line a baking pan with wax paper and place your stuffed tomatoes on top. To prevent your tomatoes from drying up too much, sprinkle a little water (about 5 tbsp). Bake tomatoes for about 25 minutes. Plate, serve and enjoy!

2. High Protein Blueberry Spinach Smoothie

SERVINGS: 2

INGREDIENTS

1 cup blueberries

2 cups baby spinach

2 Tbsp. almond butter

2 Tbsp. chia seeds

2 Tbsp. ground flaxseed

2 Tbsp. hemp seed powder

2 Tbsp. coconut oil

4 cups almond milk

PREPARATION

Blend in blueberries and spinach in almond milk, add the chia seeds, ground flaxseed, and hemp seed powder. Blend until seeds are consistent with the mixture. Add almond butter and coconut oil and blend on high to make the smoothie. Serve and enjoy! (Optional: this could be served with a little sprinkle of mint on top)

3. Minty Banana Coconut Shake

SERVINGS: 2

INGREDIENTS

2 cups coconut milk

1 cup spinach

½ cup fresh mint leaves

2 bananas, frozen

4 dates, pitted

1 tsp. vanilla

sea salt to taste

Optional: ¼ tsp. Mint extract, and/or ¼ tsp. peppermint extract

PREPARATION

Blend spinach, mint leaves, and banana into coconut milk. Make sure to thoroughly blend the spinach and mint leaves. Add in the frozen bananas and dates and blend on high. Add a teaspoon of vanilla and a small dash of sea salt to taste, mix and add more if desired. You may add in the mint and/ or peppermint extract before pouring into tall glasses. Serve and enjoy! (Optional: This fancy drink is best served with a little drizzle of chocolate flakes and coconut cream on top)

4. Lettuce Cups filled with Adzuki Beans and Avocado

SERVINGS: 2

INGREDIENTS

15-ounce can of Adzuki beans (drain and rinse)

1 avocado

1 head romaine lettuce

¼ cup minced red onion

¼ cup chopped cilantro leaves

1 lime

Sea salt to taste

Red pepper flakes (optional)

PREPARATION

In a bowl, pour in Adzuki beans and red onions and mash them together until consistent. Pour in the chopped cilantro leaves and stir until thoroughly mixed. Season with salt. Cut out romaine lettuce and form into cups. Add a spoonful of the bean and onion mash into the lettuce cups. Dice the avocado and garnish on top of the bean and onion mash. Finish with a squeeze of lime juice. Plate, serve and enjoy! (Optional: To add a little zing to every bite, sprinkle red pepper flakes before serving)

5. Lentil and Thyme Soup

SERVINGS: 4

INGREDIENTS

1 tbsp. extra virgin olive oil

1 medium onion, finely chopped

4 garlic cloves, minced

2 large carrots, chopped

2 stalks of celery, chopped

6 cups of vegetable broth

1½ cups brown lentils, rinsed

1 bay leaf

1 tsp. thyme

Small handful of parsley, chopped

Sea Salt and pepper to taste

PREPARATION

Heat a drizzle of oil in a large pot on a stove set to medium heat. Add chopped onion and fry until it turns a little brown. This will take about 5 minutes. Add carrots, garlic, and celery and fry for another 3 to 5 minutes. Mix the lentils, thyme, bay leaf into the vegetable broth and pour in the mix into the large pot. Cook soup on medium to low heat or until the lentils are tender enough. This will take about 40 minutes. Salt and pepper to taste. Stir in parsley. Serve and enjoy hot!

6. Cucumber Lavender Water

SERVINGS: 4

INGREDIENTS

1 tbsp dried lavender

8 pints water

1 medium-sized cucumber

PREPARATION

Cut cucumber into thin slices. Combine lavender, sliced cucumber and water in a pitcher and refrigerate for about half a day, or enough to let the lavender and cucumber blend in the mix. Serve and enjoy! (This is perfect for that distressing moment)

7. Watermelon Mint Water

SERVINGS: 4

INGREDIENTS

8 pints water

1 medium-sized watermelon

¼ cup mint

PREPARATION

Cut watermelon into cubed slices. Combine mint, cubed watermelon and water in a pitcher and refrigerate for about half a day, or enough to let the mint and watermelon blend in the mix. Serve and enjoy!

8. Chilled Watercress With Avocado and Cucumber Soup

SERVINGS: 2

INGREDIENTS

6 organic avocados

4 scallions

1 medium-sized cucumber

4 cups of watercress

2 lemons, freshly squeezed

3 cups of filtered water

Salt and pepper to taste

1 cup Cherry tomatoes

PREPARATION

Dice cucumber and half cherry tomatoes. Blend the cucumber, watercress, avocados, and scallions with half the water. Once the mix has turned into a thick puree pour in the rest of the water. Add lemon squeezes, salt, and pepper to taste. Continue to blend until consistent. Pour into bowls, garnish with cherry tomatoes, serve and enjoy!

9. Green Curry

SERVINGS: 4

INGREDIENTS

¼ cup coconut oil

1 large onion, peeled and diced

3 tbsp. green curry paste

1 cup green beans

1 large broccoli crown, cut into florets

1 cup snow peas

1 medium-sized Brussels sprouts, halved

4 cups garbanzo beans, cooked or canned

2 15oz. cans of unsweetened coconut milk

4 pints vegetable broth

1 bunch kale

1 bunch bok choy

Salt and pepper to taste

Fresh cilantro for garnish

PREPARATION

Drizzle large pot with coconut oil and sauté onions with curry paste until the onions are brown and tender. This will take about 10 minutes. Add green beans, broccoli, peas, Brussels sprouts, garbanzo beans and coconut milk. Combine and allow to simmer. Wait about 15 minutes. Add the vegetable broth and continue to simmer until all the vegetables have turn tender. Another 15-30 minutes. Add the kale and bok choy and season with salt and pepper. Take out of the heat. Plate with cilantro, serve and enjoy!

10. Chocolate Mousse with Avocado

SERVINGS: 2

INGREDIENTS

1½ Haas avocado

2/3 cup freshly squeezed coconut water

1 tbsp. vanilla

2 tbsp. raw cacao

3-5 dates

1½ tsp. Sea Salt

PREPARATION

Blend avocado with the coconut water until consistent. Add vanilla, cacao, and dates. Continue to blend on high. Add salt and mix. Pour, serve and enjoy!

11. Veggie Sticks with Guacamole Dip

SERVINGS: 4

INGREDIENTS:

2 avocados

2 tbsp plum tomato, finely chopped

2 tsp white onion, chopped

2 tsp freshly squeezed lime juice

2 tsp. jalapeño, diced

2 tbsp cilantro, finely chopped

2 cloves of garlic, minced

½ tsp sea salt

PREPARATION

In a bowl, mix the cilantro, onion, and jalapeño and add the salt. Using either a pestle or a large spoon, mash the ingredients together.

Add avocados to the mashed ingredients and using the pestle or a fork, mash in the avocados to the mixture. You don't have to thoroughly mash the avocados; it should just be smooth enough to blend with the ingredients but still have a little chunky texture. Stir in the finely chopped tomatoes, lime juice, and salt to taste. Serve with the mix of your veggie sticks on the side. Enjoy!

12. Naked Chilli

SERVINGS: 4

INGREDIENTS:

2 cups tomatoes, chopped

½ tsp. thyme

2 cups soaked sun-dried tomato

½ tsp thyme

½ tsp sage

1 cup cherry tomatoes

1 tsp cumin

1 tsp paprika powder

1 tsp chipotle powder

1 tsp chili powder

1 tomato, diced

¼ cup cilantro, chopped

¼ cup carrots, diced

½ cup red onion, diced

¼ cup celery, diced

¼ cup zucchini, diced

½ avocado, diced

2 garlic cloves, minced

2 scallions, diced

1 tsp jalapeño, diced

5 basil leaves, chopped

salt to taste

PREPARATION

Place all the different kinds of tomatoes into a food processor (with the "S" blade if possible) and cut for a few consecutive times. Switch the food processor to blend and add all the vegetables, as well as the garlic, jalapeño, cilantro and other powdered spices. Blend the mixture until consistent enough to liking.

Pour into a bowl and let the mixture sit for an hour. Serve with the avocado and scallions as garnish and enjoy!

13. Kale with Quinoa Salad Served with Lemon Vinaigrette Dressing

SERVINGS: 4

INGREDIENTS:

½ cup sliced almonds

½ cup pomegranate arils seeds

½ cup cooked (boiled) quinoa seeds

4 cups chopped kale

3 tbsp freshly squeezed lemon juice

¼ cup olive oil

1/4 cup apple cider vinegar

zest of lemon

PREPARATION

To prepare the dressing, whisk together the apple cider vinegar, olive oil, lemon juice and lemon zest in a small bowl and set aside.

Prepare the salad by placing the kale in a large bowl and top with quinoa, avocado, almonds and pomegranate seeds. Toss the salad (or if you want you can pour the dressing on top before tossing it, or serve with dressing on the side). Combine salad well. Salt and pepper to season. Serve and enjoy!

14. Berry Almond Smoothie

SERVINGS: 2

INGREDIENTS:

½ cup frozen strawberries

1 cup frozen blackberries

1 ½ cup almond milk

2 tbsp coconut oil

1 lime, freshly juiced

1 large bunch of kale

½ tsp vanilla

1 tbsp raw almond butter

PREPARATION

Blend in kale into the almond milk, allow to reach desired consistency. Mix in the blackberries and strawberries, coconut oil, lime, kale, vanilla and almond butter. Continue to blend until you make a smoothie. Serve in tall glasses and enjoy!

15. Banana Almond Berry Smoothie

SERVINGS: 2

INGREDIENTS:

1 frozen banana

4 tbsp raw almond butter

1 cup frozen mixed berries or strawberries

2 cups almond milk

2 cups fresh spinach

PREPARATION

Start by blending the spinach with the almond milk until you reach desired consistency. Add the banana and mixed berries or strawberries. Continue blending and add the raw almond butter. Pour smoothie into a tall glass, serve and enjoy!

16. Veggie Carrot and Leeks Soup

SERVINGS: 4

INGREDIENTS:

2 carrots

3 weeks with the green parts removed

1 thinly sliced fennel bulb

1 cup thinly sliced savoy cabbage

4 cloves minced garlic

3 tbsp coconut oil

a handful of chopped parsley

1 can kidney beans, drained and rinsed

6 cups vegetable stock

2 fresh rosemary sprigs, leaves removed and chopped

sea salt and pepper

PREPARATION

Heat a large soup pot over stove over medium-low heat. Add oil and leeks, fennel and carrots and allow vegetables to cook or until leeks are soft enough and slightly browned. This will usually take about 7 minutes.

Add the rosemary and garlic and allow to cook for another minute or so. Next, add the cabbage and sauté for another minute or two.

Pour in the vegetable stock into the mixture and allow to boil. As soon as the stock boils, add the beans and cook on low heat for about 15 minutes or until all the vegetables have gone tender.

Stir in the parsley into the soup and season with salt and pepper to taste. Pour into individual bowls, serve and enjoy!

17. Veggie Delight Pasta

SERVINGS: 4

INGREDIENTS:

1 package of kelp noodles

1 can kidney beans, drained and rinsed

1 medium head of broccoli

1 thinly sliced leek

1 spring of chopped rosemary

1 handful chopped parsley

½ tsp red pepper flakes

3 cloves minced garlic

3 tbsp extra virgin olive oil (or coconut oil)

salt and pepper

PREPARATION

Preheat oven to 400 degrees and allow to reach temperature. Toss the broccoli in garlic, red pepper flakes, extra virgin olive or coconut oil and salt. Roast the entire mix into the oven for 20 minutes or until the vegetables are tender enough upon touch with a fork.

While the vegetables are roasting, rinse and drain kelp noodles and soak in a pot filled with hot water. Meanwhile, heat 2 tablespoons of the extra virgin olive or coconut oil in a frying pan and add the leeks. Cook leeks in the pan until it has melted. This will usually take about 10 minutes.

Drain the kelp noodles and continue cooking by adding them to the melted leeks. Cook together for another 10 minutes.

Combine roasted broccoli mix into the pan. Add the parsley and rosemary. Add salt and pepper to taste in the mix.

Mix in the kidney beans. Plate in a salad bowl, serve and enjoy!

18. Brussels Sprouts Salad with Pistachios and Lemon

SERVINGS: 4

INGREDIENTS:

16 large Brussels sprouts (end of the sprout cut off and leaves peeled off from the core)

¾ cup shelled pistachios

zest and juice collected from one lemon

2 tbsp. extra virgin olive oil

salt and pepper to taste

PREPARATION

Drizzle oil on a large skillet or wok and place on top of the stove to heat on medium-high for a few minutes. Add the pistachios to the skillet (or wok) and the lemon zest. Sauté mix for an entire minute before you add the Brussels Sprouts leaves. Toss the mix until Brussels sprouts are bright green enough but still crisp. This will take about 5 minutes.

Squeeze lemon juice over the mixture. Toss and season with salt and pepper. Plate in a salad bowl, serve and enjoy!

19. Pasta Zucchini with Spinach Lemon Pesto

SERVINGS: 2

INGREDIENTS:

4 zucchinis

3 cups baby spinach

Juice of 1 small to medium lemon

½ cup cherry tomatoes, sliced in half

½ cup extra-virgin olive oil

¼ cup cashews

3 garlic cloves

¼ cup basil

PREPARATION

Using a spiralizer, make zucchini pasta by making it into long strands. This is best done using raw zucchini or flash sautéed for two minutes.

Meanwhile, in a food processor with an "S" blade, mix in spinach, garlic, basil and cashews, and pulse until finely chopped. Keep the food processor on and slowly add in the lemon juice and olive oil.

Season with salt and pepper to taste.

Toss the freshly prepared zucchini pasta and spinach lemon pesto together. Garnish the dish with cherry tomatoes. Plate in a large salad bowl, serve and enjoy!

20. Sweet Potato Soup With a Hint of Curry

SERVINGS: 4

INGREDIENTS:

3 peeled sweet potatoes, cut into 1-inch cubes

2 tsp. curry

2 cups water

1 15oz can of full-fat coconut milk

zest and juice of one lime

4 cloves garlic, minced

1 ½ inch piece of ginger, sliced and crushed

1 tbs. coconut oil

½ bunch cilantro, chopped

PREPARATION

In a large saucepan, add coconut oil and heat pan on the stove over medium heat. Add the garlic, ginger and lime zest and cook until the garlic is slightly browned. This will take about 5 minutes.

Add curry to the pan and cook until fragrant. Normally takes another minute.

Stir in coconut milk and water along with sweet potatoes. Bring mixture to a boil and reduce to low and simmer. Cover for about 25 more minutes and allow to simmer.

Turn the heat off and leave the pot on the stove for about a half hour to allow flavors to blend.

Using a blender or a food processor, puree the soup. Garnish the final puree with chopped cilantro and dash with lime juice.

Serve in a bowl and enjoy!

21. Alkaline Power Up Treats

SERVINGS: 3

INGREDIENTS:

1 cup hulled hemp seeds

2 tsp vanilla

3 tsp cinnamon

¼ cup cacao nibs

3 tsp chia seeds

¼ cup flax seeds

6 pitted dates

1 cup raw almond butter

PREPARATION

Mix in the a processor the cup of raw almond butter and six pitted dates.

Add the rest of the remaining ingredients into the food processor except for the hemp seeds. Continue pulsing until you have created a ball in the food processor.

Using your hands, roll mix into inch-sized balls and then coat the treats in hemp seeds as well as the 3 teaspoons of chia seeds.

Store the balls in an airtight container. These treats are good for up to a week. Plate on a plate, serve and enjoy!

22. Choco Mint Smoothie

SERVINGS: 2

INGREDIENTS:

1 cup of frozen coconut water

1 tsp chia seeds

½ small avocado

½ cup packed mint leaves

2 tbsp cacao nibs

1 cup almond milk

4 pitted dates

¼ cup raw almonds

PREPARATION

Start by blending the coconut water ice with the cup of almond milk and avocado scoops. Add the rest of the mint leaves, cacao nibs and dates. Pulse until you have created a smoothie. Pour into tall glass, garnish with chia seeds, serve and enjoy!

23. Detoxifying Ginger Lemon Turmeric Tea

SERVINGS: 2

INGREDIENTS:

1 lemon slice

pinch of black pepper

1 inch of fresh organic ginger root

1 inch of fresh organic turmeric root

about 20 oz water

PREPARATION

Bring water in a pot to a boil. While the water is boiling, peel the turmeric and ginger and dice them into small pieces. The size would depend on your preference for taste, the smaller the dices, the more flavourful the tea would be.

Once the water has boiled, remove the pot of water from the heat and add turmeric, ginger and black pepper to the pot. Replace pot on the stove and simmer for another 10 minutes. This again would depend on how strong you would want the tea. The more you simmer, the stronger the flavor.

Pour into a cup and serve with a squeeze of lemon. Leftovers can be stored in an airtight container in the fridge and can be served as iced tea. Enjoy!

Conclusion

Whether it is to improve your weight or reduce your risk of developing all the diseases and disorders that are associated with metabolic acidosis, or that condition where your body's pH is below the optimal range. Your decision to ditch the high fat, simple sugar diet and switch to the high alkalinity inducing one is probably the best favor you have done your body just yet.

As you have seen throughout the book, and as we have continued to emphasize and justify in the book, backed up with a lot of scientific research and real-life practical claims. The alkaline diet is definitely for you! It does not matter whether you are a fully pledged stay at home mom, or a hardworking young male professional with the stead nine to five routine. Or a recovering cancer survivor or a senior citizen with some struggles with chronic muscle pains, then the alkaline diet can be your solution to achieving the body and health you have been striving for. It does not even matter how young you are, because as it shows you are never too young to enter into the alkaline diet. There are no restrictions or limitations.

I hope that this book has helped encourage you to dive into the alkaline diet and sooner experience all the benefits associated with this beautiful not so secret.

And as a parting gesture, we salute and congratulate you on your journey towards self-growth, improved health and better lifestyle.

Final Words

Thank you again for purchasing this book!

I really hope this book is able to help you.

The next step is for you to **join our email newsletter** to receive updates on any upcoming new book releases or promotions. You can sign-up for free and as a bonus, you will also receive our "*7 Fitness Mistakes You Don't Know You're Making*" book! This bonus book breaks down many of the most common fitness mistakes and will demystify many of the complexities and science of getting into shape. Having all this fitness knowledge and science organized into an actionable step-by-step book will help you get started in the right direction in your fitness journey! To join our free email newsletter and grab your free book, please visit the link and signup: **www.hmwpublishing.com/gift**

Finally, if you enjoyed this book, then I would like to ask you for a favor, would you be kind enough to leave a review for this book? It would be greatly appreciated!

Thank you and good luck in your journey!

About the Co-Author

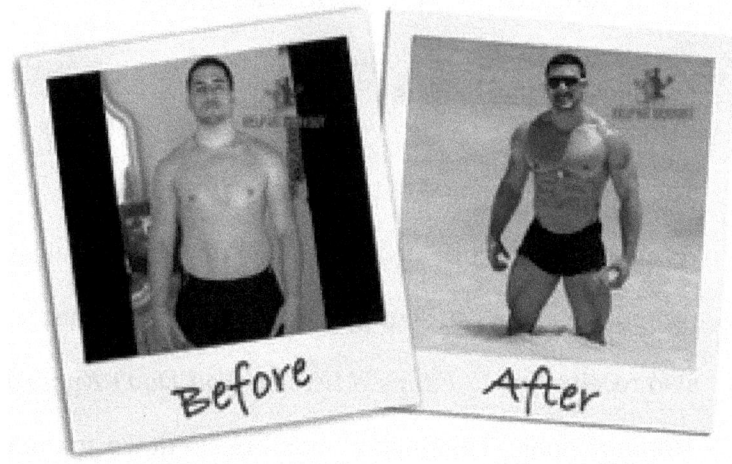

My name is George Kaplo; I'm a certified personal trainer from Montreal, Canada. I'll start off by saying I'm not the biggest guy you will ever meet and this has never really been my goal. In fact, I started working out to overcome my biggest insecurity when I was younger, which was my self-confidence. This was due to my height measuring only 5 foot 5 inches (168cm), it pushed me down to attempt anything I ever wanted to achieve in life. You may be going through some challenges right now, or you may simply want to get fit, and I can certainly relate.

For me personally, I was always kind of interested in the health & fitness world and wanted to gain some muscle due to the numerous bullying in my teenage years about my height and my overweight body. I figured I couldn't do anything about my height, but I sure can do something about how my body looked like. This was the beginning of my transformation journey. I had no idea where to start, but I just got started. I felt worried and afraid at times that other people would make fun of me for doing the exercises the wrong way. I always wished I had a friend that was next to me who was knowledgeable enough to help me get started and "show me the ropes."

After a lot of work, studying and countless trial and errors. Some people began to notice how I was getting more fit and how I was starting to form a keen interest in the topic. This led many friends and new faces to come to me and ask me for fitness advice. At first, it seemed odd when people asked me to help them get in shape. But what kept me going is when they started to see changes in their own body and told me it's the first time that they saw real results! From there, more people kept coming to me, and it made me realize after so much reading and studying in this field that it did help me but it also allowed me to help others. I'm now a fully certified personal trainer and have trained numerous clients to date who have achieved amazing results.

Today, my brother Alex Kaplo (also a Certified Personal Trainer) and I own & operate this publishing venture, where we bring passionate and expert authors to write about health and fitness topics. We also run an online fitness website "HelpMeWorkout.com" and I would love to connect with by inviting you to visit the website on the following page and signing up to our e-mail newsletter (you will even get a free book).

Last but not least, if you are in the position I was once in and you want some guidance, don't hesitate and ask... I'll be there to help you out!

Your friend and coach,

George Kaplo
Certified Personal Trainer

Get another book for Free

I want to thank you for purchasing this book and offer you another book (just as long and valuable as this book), "Health & Fitness Mistakes You Don't Know You're Making", completely free.

Visit the link below to signup and receive it:

www.hmwpublishing.com/gift

In this book, I will break down the most common health & fitness mistakes, you are probably committing right now, and I will reveal how you can easily get in the best shape of your life!

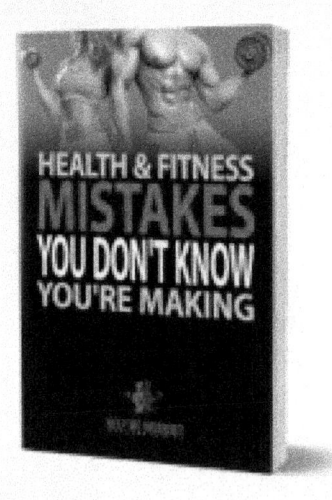

In addition to this valuable gift, you will also have an opportunity to get our new books for free, enter giveaways, and receive other valuable emails from me. Again, visit the link to sign up:

www.hmwpublishing.com/gift

Copyright 2017 by HMW Publishing - All Rights Reserved.

This document by HMW Publishing owned by the A&G Direct Inc company, is geared towards providing exact and reliable information in regards to the topic and issue covered. The publication is sold with the idea that the publisher is not required to render accounting, officially permitted, or otherwise, qualified services. If advice is necessary, legal or professional, a practiced individual in the profession should be ordered.

From a Declaration of Principles which was accepted and approved equally by a Committee of the American Bar Association and a Committee of Publishers and Associations.

In no way is it legal to reproduce, duplicate, or transmit any part of this document in either electronic means or in printed format. Recording of this publication is strictly prohibited, and any storage of this document is not allowed unless with written permission from the publisher. All rights reserved.

The information provided herein is stated to be truthful and consistent, in that any liability, in terms of inattention or otherwise, by any usage or abuse of any policies, processes, or directions contained within is the solitary and utter responsibility of the recipient reader. Under no circumstances will any legal responsibility or blame be held against the publisher for any reparation, damages, or monetary loss due to the information herein, either directly or indirectly.

The information herein is offered for informational purposes solely, and is universal as so. The presentation of the information is without contract or any type of guarantee assurance.

The trademarks that are used are without any consent, and the publication of the trademark is without permission or backing by the trademark owner. All trademarks and brands within this book are for clarifying purposes only and are the owned by the owners themselves, not affiliated with this document.

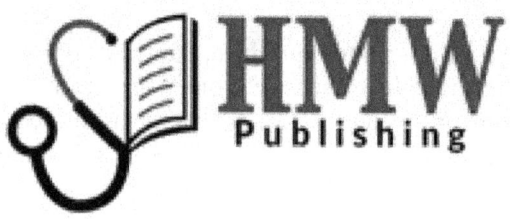

For more great books visit:

HMWPublishing.com

www.ingramcontent.com/pod-product-compliance
Lightning Source LLC
Chambersburg PA
CBHW071113030426
42336CB00013BA/2059